Clean Eating Recipes & Menu Plan: Simple and Easy Menu Plan with Delicious Clean Eating Recipes

Rediscover Your Body's Natural Balance and Ability to Heal With Clean Eating Diet & Menu Plan

By: Barbara Neil

PUBLISHERS NOTES

This publication is intended to provide helpful and informative material. It is not intended to diagnose, treat, cure, or prevent any health problem or condition, nor is intended to replace the advice of a physician. No action should be taken solely on the contents of this book. Always consult your physician or qualified health-care professional on any matters regarding your health and before adopting any suggestions in this book or drawing inferences from it.

The author and publisher specifically disclaim all responsibility for any liability, loss or risk, personal or otherwise, which is incurred as a consequence, directly or indirectly, from the use or application of any contents of this book.

Always read all information provided by the manufacturers' product labels before using their products. The author and publisher are not responsible for claims made by manufacturers.

Table of Contents

DEDICATION

This book is dedicated to my mentor for making this book possible in all aspects.

INTRODUCTION

Even at the beginning of life, man has to depend on food to supplement life. Food plays an important role in the very existence of man. It provides the human body with energy, supplies the materials necessary for its growth and maintenance, and furnishes various substances essentials for it to properly function.

All of these are met by the constituents of food or known as nutrients, the most important of which are fats, carbohydrates, proteins, minerals, and vitamins. The health of the body is very much dependent on the amount and quality of nutrients the body takes from its diet.

Along with the industrial revolution, there are many changes in the way man handles food. Food preservation, canning, and further food processes were introduced. These developments in food handling have given flexibility for man to store food, however, the nutrients that the body needs are lost if not minimally retained. The health of man has declined a great deal. It is in this regard that professional food handlers have come to reintroduce the concept of clean eating.

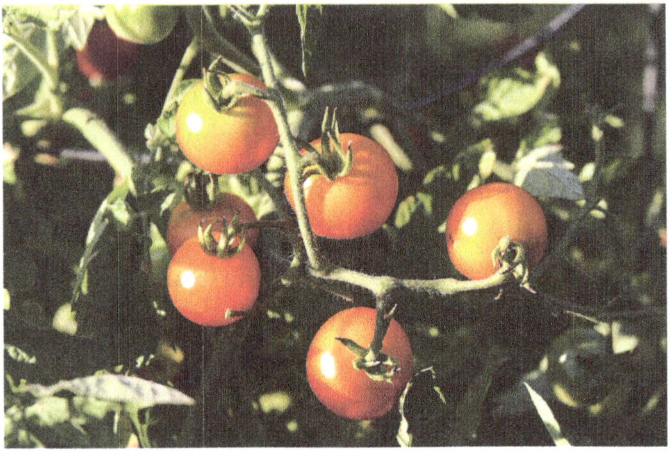

What is Clean Eating?

Clean eating is basically going back to the source of food. It is the consumption of food as close to its original state. An example: the consumption of fresh potatoes versus potato chips, or the consumption of fresh fish versus canned sardines. This brings any aspiring clean eater to go back to the natural source of food.

Sources of food

All food comes from plants and animals. Foods of vegetable origin include cereals, starchy roots and tubers (underground stems), pulses (seeds of pod-bearing plants), nuts, fruits, and vegetables. Among those of animal origin are meat, milk, poultry, eggs, and fish. Fats and oils may be either vegetable or animal origin.

The concept of clean eating can be used to correct the growing problems of obesity, heart problems, diabetes, and other diseases. Clean eating is more likely to go by the rule of prevention over cure. Whatever you feed your body, your body will react in the form of good health.

Good health means high resistance to diseases. It is in this concept that clean eating is important as a basis to arrange the perfect healthy meals for the whole family. It offers the required nutrition, while keeping away unnecessary growth and accumulation of harmful substances in the body. Clean eating can be practiced as one of the best remedy for enjoying longer and a healthier life.

CHAPTER 1
-
What is clean eating?

What does it mean to eat clean?

Eating clean means that you are eating foods that are as close to their natural state as possible. This also means eating whole foods, not the grocery store whole foods, but foods that are in their whole state.

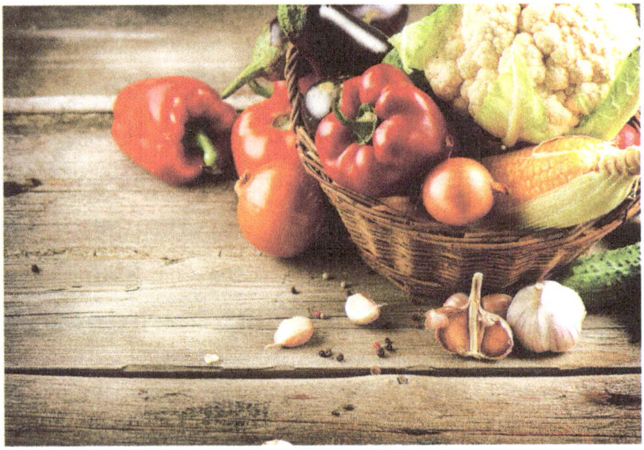

Clean eating comprises of foods that are prepared with only a single or a couple of ingredients. Examples of these are consuming plain bananas with no other additives or consuming just Kale and no other ingredients added.

The basic rule of thumb in clean eating is that if the food spoils rather quickly, like less than a month or so, then it is healthier for the body (this rule may not be always be true).

On the other hand, when foods are kept in a box, it may not be healthy because of the high possibility of added preservatives. It is always good to take note that packaged foods can be tricky and may claim it to be healthy because of its commercial nature.

Foods that are served fresh and in its natural state are the best food choices for clean eating.

Organic or Non organic

Clean eating can also mean consuming foods that are organic or locally grown. There are a few questions raised with regards to a choice of organic foods, "Do I always have to get organic?" or "Why do you always have to choose organic?" Organic is great because you are getting rid of all the pesticides and stuff that they spray on the fruits and veggies.

You do not want these chemicals in your body.

Ingesting these chemicals unknowingly can really make you feel bad or even cause damage to your whole system and, thus, your health can be jeopardized.

Organic is always a good choice, however, there are other foods that can be exempt from being organic.

Foods exempt from being organic:

- Choosing fruits like watermelon and banana, which really has a thick layer of skin, need not be organic. The thick peel of these fruits protect the inner layer from possible pesticides sprayed into it and, therefore, can still be safe for eating.
- Fruits and vegetables with a really thin peel like apples, grapes, bell peppers, and carrots are usually eaten with skin. Choosing organic is best for these types of fruits and vegetables.
- Green and leafy vegetables are best to be organic because you are actually eating the leaf; you are not really peeling off anything to get the good stuff.

Processed over Unprocessed Foods

Eating clean can also mean eating foods that are unprocessed. Some examples of these are fruits, veggies, and whole grains that are not processed. Oatmeal, for example, can become tricky because some oatmeal products are processed. Going for raw oatmeal would be the best option. You want to try the steel cut oats because they are more natural than the processed version of oats.

Anything in a box or packaged are most likely processed. If it is made in a factory or a person created it with chemicals to preserve the food, don't eat it. Keep it out of your diet as much as possible. As far as clean eating is concerned, go for unprocessed foods.

Stay especially away from cartons of juice that says it is made with real juice, this has a whole bunch of sugar, chemicals, and preservatives added that you just want to keep out of your body. These ingredients can cause inflammation in your mid-section, which is very unhealthy for your body.

Here a few good choices of unprocessed foods:

- Freshly Squeezed Juice. Juicing is great because it actually breaks down the fruit or vegetable and then extracts all the great nutrients, minerals, and vitamins that are essential to the body.
- Whole Grains. Incorporate unprocessed whole grains into your diet like brown rice, millet, and quinoa, which are rich in protein. Choose steel cut oats over processed oats. Steel cut oats are round and harder while processed oats are flat in texture. Unprocessed oats also take longer to cook, but they are much better for you.
- Lean Meat, Chicken and Fish. Lean meats are meats that have more muscles than fats. While lean meat and chicken are good, fish like salmon is amazing! It is high in omega 3 fatty acids, which are great for reducing inflammation that you can get around your mid-section.
- Grass fed poultry and meat are a better choice over farm raised cattle and poultry. Farm raised cattle and poultry become fatty because they are not freely raised in the open. If you can, check to make sure that they are grass-fed, meaning that they are fed

a more plant based diet.

- Avoid Processed Sugars. White sugar is a processed sugar. The sugar in bananas and fruits like apples or oranges are natural and totally fine for the body. But anything that is high in sugar like soda and candy are bad sugar and it should be kept out of your diet.
- Avoid Hydrogenated Saturated fats. While there are natural fats that are good for the body, such as those coming from coconut oil, a process called hydrogenation is an artificial manipulation of fats that push natural oils to a saturated state by adding hydrogen atoms. This process benefits processed food shelf life, but is not healthy for the body.

If you are craving for something sweet, a good recommendation is a good fruit salad. Get a whole bunch of raspberries, blueberries, kiwi, and bananas. Chop them into small pieces, put it together, and toss like a salad. It is really good when you have a sweet tooth at nighttime.

This salad skips all the additives and preservatives that are really bad for you. Choose lean cuts of meat and get your content more from nuts, fish, avocado, organic peanut butter, and other fruits and vegetables that have all the good nutrients in them.

Clean Eating and a Vegan Lifestyle

Clean eating is not suggestive of being a vegetarian or switching to a vegan lifestyle. While clean eating enthusiasts are appreciative of a vegan lifestyle, they still opt to add some controlled amounts of lean meat and dairy products to their diet.

A person who follows a strict clean eating lifestyle would totally take out dairy products in their diet, such as milk, cheese, and anything that has dairy in it. However, strict clean eating still includes lean meat, fish, and chicken to their diet, which does not qualify them to be labeled vegetarians. Clean eating is getting the right nutrition and keeping a clean and healthy diet.

Clean Eating To Alkalize Your Body

When all of the bad stuff from processed foods is absorbed in the body, it accumulates in the intestinal area, which causes inflammation and increases acidity. To remove acid buildup, a person would want to alkalize the body by incorporating a lot of fresh fruits and veggies in their diet. Parsley and Cilantro are two mini leafy greens that are great for alkalizing the body, reducing the acidity, which causes the inflammation.

CHAPTER 2
-
Essential Benefits of Clean Eating

Fact: In the United States of America alone, the growing number of obesity problems has been very alarming in recent years. Figures show that more than 35% of American adults are diagnosed with being obese. In 2011, the obesity rate among adults exceeded 30% in just twelve states while 27 states are now pouncing on 25% in adult obesity.

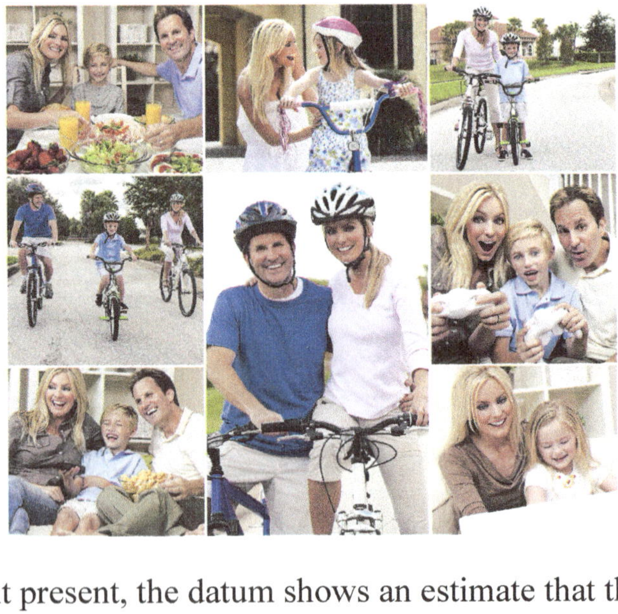

At present, the datum shows an estimate that the

rate of obesity among adults can hit or exceed 44% in all states by the year 2030.

The fact sheet of obesity is alarming. To think that this is just one disease that man has to deal with. Cancer is a growing problem, not to mention diabetes and other diseases, which leads to high death rates due to sickness. Although there are possible cures to these ailments, it is always better to prevent than to cure.

Many food experts have gone back to man's food intake to have a huge contribution to prevent diseases from even occurring. Man has to rediscover Clean Eating, doing away with processed foods and embracing natural foods as close to its original state as possible.

The Clean Eating Concept

- The basic form of food should be eaten. The clean eater must find food in its natural form. It may be vegetables, fruits, eggs, or meat (Healthy fats and lean protein).
- Refrain from processed and artificial food. The clean eater must stop or minimize the consummation of processed or genetically

modified food items.

- The labels should be read very carefully in the practice of clean eating. The food items with a long ingredient list should be avoided.
- Get away from processed or refined food, such as pasta, noodles, white sugar, and even iodized salt.
- The selection of food must be done in a very careful manner. The fruits and vegetables from organic farms and flesh of naturally raised animals should be selected.
- A person must consume plenty of water. It is better to have 2 liters per day, and the consumption of alcoholic beverages and other types of soft drinks should be minimized or even stopped.
- The quantity of serving per meal must be reduced and the number of meals per day should be increased. It helps to supply the food as it burns down. It is better to have three meals and three snacks per day.

Benefits of Eating Clean

With the concept of clean eating, there is a good chance of increasing quality nutrients into the body; at the same time, removing junk from the system while water flushes out other impurities. Clean eating increases the body's stamina and strengthens the body's natural immune system.

The 6-meal plan

Many people, who are new to this concept, will be amazed at the number of meals that have to be taken per day. In the process of clean eating the number of meals per day is higher, but the food serving becomes smaller. The food serving per meal should be enough to supply the energy and the nutritional needs of the body.

In the normal three-meal system, there is a certain period that the body has to be without food to supply energy, so it is not a suitable situation. The time gap between 2 meals is about 2-3 hours in the clean eating process, and the amount of food is just enough for the body. So there will be no excess or lack of food in the stomach and, thus, there will not be any threat of gastritis and diabetes.

Consuming lean protein and complex carbohydrate

Complex carbohydrates such as whole grain, vegetables, and fruits can be more beneficial than the simple carbohydrates like white rice and bread. Complex carbohydrates have more nutrients and it takes more time to digest, which is very beneficial to people who are suffering from diabetes. Lean protein comes from animal sources; therefore, there is less chance of saturated fats.

Two servings of healthy fats daily (unsaturated)

Fat is an essential nutrient for the human body and it comes from various sources such as butter, margarine, meat, fish, and etc. However, the issue of cholesterol is a concern when taken in excessive amounts. Cholesterol has become a great health issue in the United States and other countries in the world, tracing back the cause to increased consumption of fatty meat in various forms. In this regard, it is at its best to minimize fats in any daily dietary plan.

Fresh vegetables and fruits

There are several benefits of taking fruits and vegetables. It offers potassium, dietary fiber, and vitamin C. Fruits and vegetables have no issues in high cholesterol, excessive sugar, or fats. Therefore, these foods are the best contributory sources for quality nutrients. Dietary fiber found in fresh fruits and vegetables can reduce blood cholesterol levels and minimize heart diseases. Vitamin c is very important to the growth and repair of body tissues. Folate (folic acid) is responsible for producing red blood cells, so it is essential to the body, specifically for expecting mothers.

Food in smaller servings

Obesity has become a social issue in many countries. One of the reasons is excessive eating of trendy processed foods. The "smaller serving" concept of clean eating can help discipline the body to have the right energy it needs throughout the day.

Increased water intake

Water hydrates the body and rejuvenates the body cells. Apart from hydration, water has the capability to flush out all impurities in the body in the form of urine and feces.

CHAPTER 3
-
Importance of Water in Clean Eating

Water is the life of the human world. Water covers almost every aspect of the environment. The body consists of a large amount of water in several structures. It is extremely helpful in several functions of the body. The human body is composed of 60% of water.

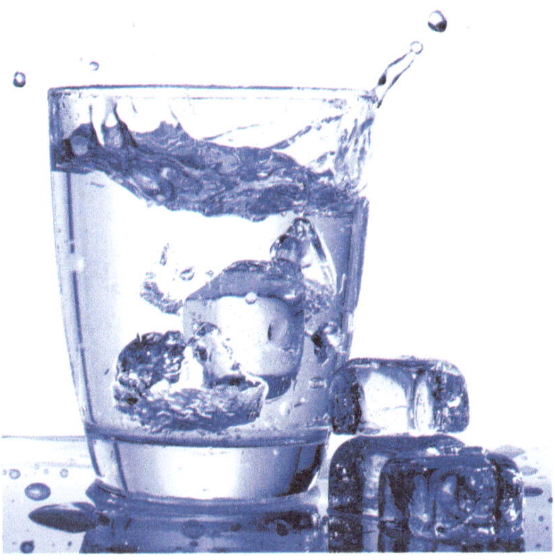

The brain is made up of about 94% of water, and lungs contain about 82% of water.

Generally, the importance of water is great. Regular intake of liquids is essential to maintain the right body functions. In the process of clean eating, water has the biggest role in place.

Nutrition experts reiterate the importance of consuming 8 glasses of water in a day. Liquids in the form of fruit juices are a great addition to water to complete the required daily water supplement of the body. An average adult male should maintain about 3 liters of liquids, while children and females should take 2.2 liters. Clean eating emphasizes that the higher amount of fluid intake must come from water. Pure water is very beneficial in the process of clean eating.

If there is a loss of more than 2% of water, there will be signs of dehydration. Estimates show that more than 75% Americans are in mild chronic dehydration condition. This is a very critical issue, as there are several adverse effects on this. Clean eating practice can be a good solution because of its high regard in drinking water as part of the eating practice.

Water is pretty basic in all of the activities in the human body. It regulates good digestion, absorption, transportation, and circulation of nutrients. It helps the body produce saliva and other forms of liquids needed in the body. It also helps maintain the right temperature of the body.

Water as a lubricant

Water is a lubricating agent in several processes of the body. During the clean eating process, a lot of attention is given to the consumption of various types of fresh fruits and vegetables. While in the process of the digestion, lots of water is needed for better digestion.

Water creates saliva, which helps to chew and swallow foods. Water in the walls of the esophagus lets the food slide down to the stomach easily. Clean eating supports the consumption of whole grains and a lot of fruits and vegetables, so a large amount of water is needed in the process.

Water removes harmful toxins

There are more than 8000 identified toxins, which affect the human body. Some enter from the environment and others are created by the body itself. The removal of these toxins must be done in order to keep the body in perfect condition.

Water can remove toxins in several ways. It removes several toxins by urination and perspiration. Water helps move waste from the large intestines and out of the body while at the same time helps maintain moisture throughout the intestinal walls. The high intake of water in the clean eating process can improve the functions of the kidney and the liver.

Water maintains various bodily functions

The efficiency of all bodily processes can improve by consuming lots of water. Blood is responsible for all the transportation of nutrients throughout the body and blood is composed of 92% water.

The food is digested and turned into water-soluble nutrients. These nutrients shall be transported to various parts of the body. These nutrients pass through the blood to the circulatory system with the help of water.

Prevention of diseases

Cancer has become a critical social issue. To help cancer patients in their journey to wellness and as prevention, water therapy is advised for the majority of patients suffering from cancer. Certain types of cancer, such as colon cancer, are advised to considerably increase intake of water. It is estimated that drinking more water can reduce about 45% of colon cancers and 50% of bladder cancers.

Water helps regulate body temperature

Water plays a very important role in maintaining and controlling body temperature. The human body has a precise temperature to maintain in order to keep the metabolic activity function in the right manner. The heat from the outside can affect the functions of the body and can really be harmful.

Water refreshes the exterior of the body and in turn brings the temperature down. Heat is also regulated by the help of perspiration. Notice that when the body is exhausted and in heat, the body automatically releases sweat. This is because the body automatically reacts to regulate body temperature.

Water enhances the appearance

Water rejuvenates and refreshes the skin. It helps maintain its elasticity and at the same time naturally moisturizes it. It is also water that helps improve the condition of your hair, as it naturally moisturizes the scalp as it does the skin.

CHAPTER 4
-
Clean Eating Diet Plan for the Whole Family

Clean eating encourages people to eat more and more nutritious food. The idea does not suggest a person to be a vegetarian; it is simply refraining from certain food items that are artificial and synthetic. One who decides to follow the clean eating procedure must follow a simple rule:

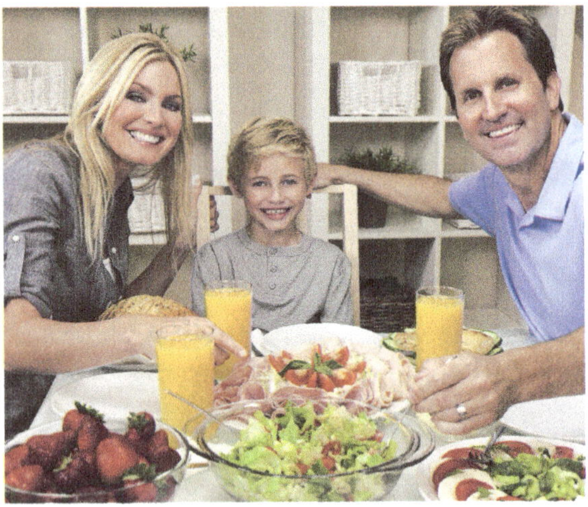

Being able to find nutritious and tasty food types in their almost natural form. Fruits, vegetables, and lean meats are the basic food types that will compose most of the family meals.

A better understanding of the food types is helpful to plan a nutritious, yet clean meal. The GO, Grow, and Glow foods are the food items you want to get in its natural form. The trick to follow a successful meal plan is to start simple – plan, shop, and prepare!

Understanding the food pyramid

The food pyramid is a great guide to outline the right foods to prepare every day. Understanding the food group within the pyramid will make clean eating meal planning so much easier. Let's take a look at the whole picture.

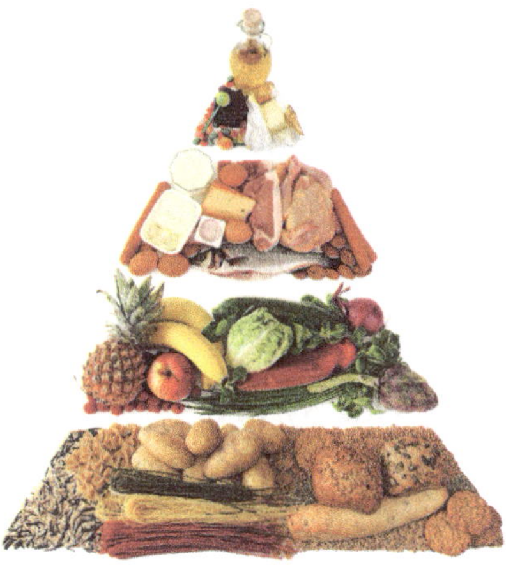

Energy Foods

The base of the pyramid composes the largest part of the pyramid, which is the energy foods, meaning you need the most servings from this food group daily, which is at 6-11 servings per day. This food groups are as follows: foods from grains, breads, cereal, and rice.

Vitamins and Minerals

The second level from the base is composed of fruits and vegetables, which are rich in vitamins, minerals, and fiber. They come next in the most servings, which are ideally 3-5 servings for vegetables and 2-4 servings for fruits.

Protein Foods

The third from the base is the protein group of foods, which are composed of foods mostly coming from animals. This includes milk, yogurt, and cheese; meats, poultry, fish, dried beans, and eggs. Nuts are included in this food group because of its high protein content. The recommended serving is 2-3 per day.

Healthy Fats and Sweets

The tip of the pyramid is composed of healthy fats, oils, and sweets. These are foods that are usually added in salad dressings such as butter, mayonnaise, and margarine. These types of food should be used sparingly.

These facts will be very helpful for a beginner to plan a clean eating diet. At the beginning, it will not be an easy task, but through time, you will be able to create the most appropriate diet plans for the family without much trouble. The meal guide is very useful for planning a clean eating meal.

Here is a starter sample meal plan that you can use and personalize. What you will see here are general meals that you can adapt for breakfast, lunch, and dinner.

Sample Meal Plan

Breakfast (one week plan):

- Pancakes
- Porridge
- Pudding
- Vegetable/Fruit Shake
- Mixed Fruits
- Raw Cereals
- Smoothies

Lunch (one week plan):

- Fruit or vegetable salad
- Steamed Chicken/Grilled lean meat
- Black beans and grilled steak
- Beef, onion and lentil salad
- Loaded Quinoa bowl
- Vegetable Chili
- Caesar Salad

Dinner (one week plan):

- Salmon, squash fries and botchy or rice rolls and vegetables
- Spinach and chicken salad or potato chicken salad
- Vegetable lasagna/pasta servings
- Vegetarian burrito/ mushroom soup
- Brown rice and stir fry vegetable mix
- Mini steak and vegetable pizza
- Mushroom Soup and wheat bread

To get you started with a clean eating diet, it is always nice to start by shopping for the right foods and placing those in your cart. Fruits and vegetables are always a good source to start clean eating; rice, raw cereals, and eggs are the simplest food items to add to your shopping list. Always check the label when shopping.

Get started with your shopping list

Instead of

- White sugar
- White bread
- Dairy fat
- Baked sweets
- Processed meats

Try

- Brown sugar
- Wheat bread
- Low-fat versions
- homemade cookies or bars
- Freshly cut lean meat, fish, skinless chicken

Getting started may be overwhelming, but it is always easy, as long as the meal plan is kept simple. Shakes are always an easy way to get through the morning meals, salad and mashed potatoes at lunch, and soup in the evening. This is ideal for those who live solo.

But to those who have a family to include in the meal planning, go for pancakes and pudding in the morning, use shakes in between meals, protein rich meals at lunch, and you may go vegetarian with soup in the evening.

The energy giving foods are very important. You may have carbohydrates like rice, pasta, or cereals for breakfast and lunch, but it is most ideal to have less at dinner, but intake more protein. Shakes in the morning and soup in the evening is a nice and effective plan I always follow.

Fruits and vegetables are ideal at any part of your meal; you can have them for breakfast, lunch, or dinner or for all of your meals in a day. Nevertheless, a balanced meal is always important, so try to spread out the need for carbohydrates and protein in your planning.

For your shakes and smoothies, you can grab dozens of fruit and vegetable smoothies for morning meals and snack time. Fruits are usually easier to prepare and are more acceptable by the whole family, especially for kids. In between your meal planning, it is good to add a full glass of water before meals and another glass of water after. This helps the digestive system move out waste in the morning.

Find a healthy clean eating recipe to get an idea of what to pick up the next time you go to the grocery store. These healthy recipes are meals that are already pre-planned and just need to be prepared. Getting a good set of clean eating recipe books will complete a week of clean eating meals.

Gradual change is necessary. You do not have to let your family jump into the 6-meal plan all at once. You can follow the 3-day meal plan for 3 days and then jump into a 4-day meal plan for another 3 days, then to a 5-day meal plan for another 3 days until you will be well adjusted to the 6-day meal plan.

Don't expect to get it right the first time. Preparing a perfect meal plan will take months to master and manage. Gradual change is necessary. It can be done in a very slow but careful manner. A simple change can be very helpful in creating a great result in the diet, as an example, a salad can be added to the list. One by one a new food type can be introduced to the list.

CHAPTER 5
-
Complete Clean Eating Meal

Many in every nook and corner of the world have followed this clean eating process. There are no restrictions or strict limitations of certain food items, as most of the other dieting methods follow.

In the process of clean eating, the restrictions are very few, and there are lots of options to make the meal attractive and delicious. Usually the clean eating process should consist of 5 to 6 meals. The portions and the types are arranged according to the need of the energy for the body. Given below is a clean eating meal plan, and this is a perfect meal plan for a day. There are 6 meals.

First meal: Peanut butter with oatmeal

This is the main part of the first meal, and it offers the energy and the other types of the nutrients to start the day and to maintain the energy to perform other activities.

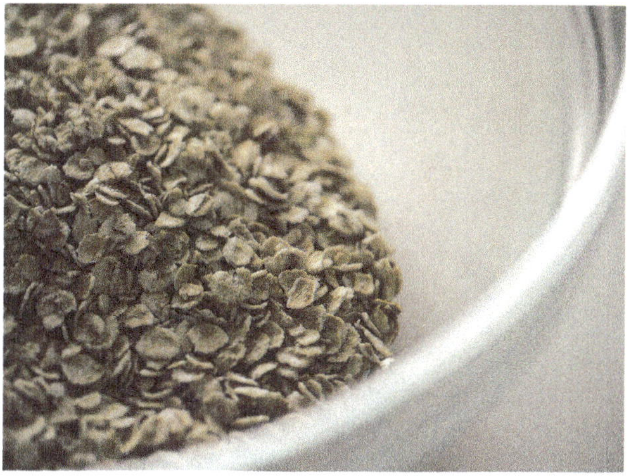

Ingredients

- I -1/2 cups of cooked oats (It can be cooked with almond milk or coconut milk)
- 2 ½ tablespoons of fresh almond butter
- 1 teaspoon of cinnamon
- 1-2 tablespoons of honey
- (2 eggs are added during the process of cooking)

How to make?

First, take a saucepan and let the oats warm, then put the warm oats into a bowl and add all other ingredients, then mix it well until they are totally combined with each other.

Second meal: A pear and some juicy fruits

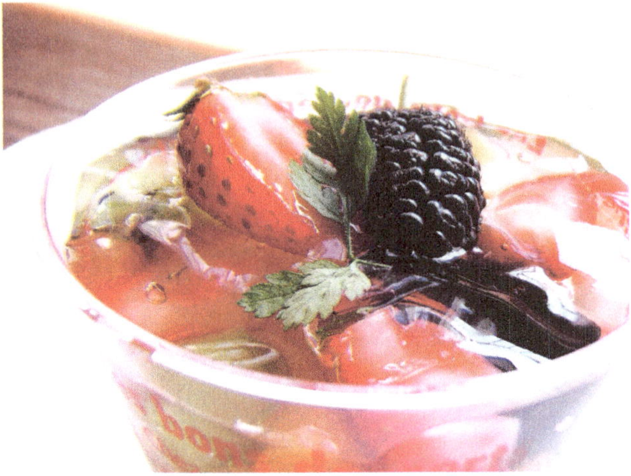

A farm fresh pear and some grapes and bananas can be taken. The amount of the fruits should not be higher than 2 cups.

Third meal: Berry smoothie and some nuts

A delicious Berry smoothie will do a great service for the third meal of the day.

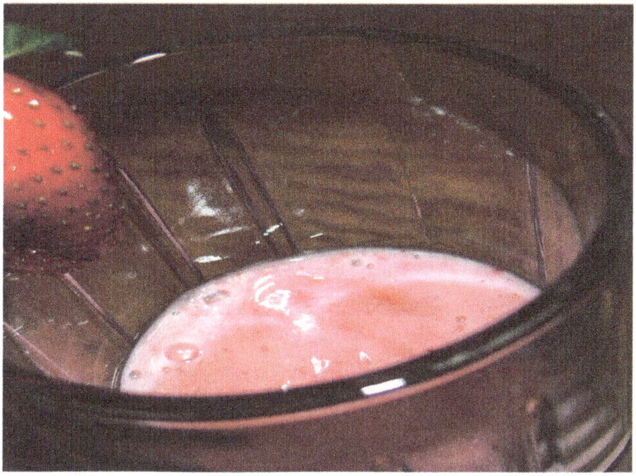

Ingredients

- 1 Cup of Kefir
- 1 cup of strawberries
- 1-2 tablespoons of honey

How to make?

- Place the Kefir in the blender
- Then add in the strawberries and honey
- Blend it until it reaches a very smooth consistency

Fourth meal: Turkey chili and 2 slices of corn bread

The Turkey chili can be very tasty, as well as a nutritious dish, this recipe is for 8 people and it will take 1 and half hours to complete.

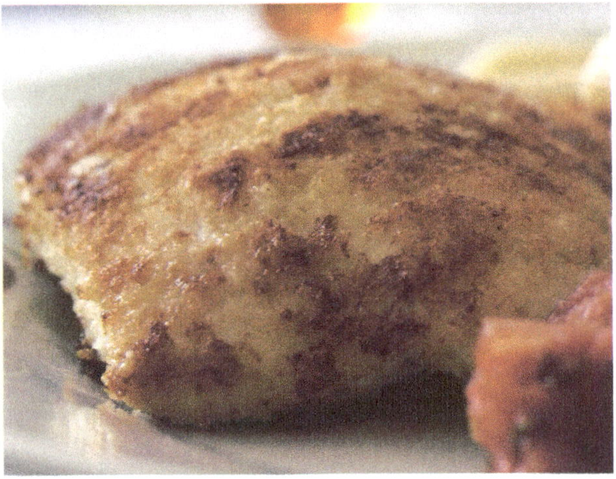

Ingredients

- 1 tablespoons of vegetable oil (unsaturated)
- 1 1/2 pounds of properly ground turkey
- 2 cups of roughly chopped onion
- 2 1/2 tablespoons of fine chili powder
- 1 tablespoon of thinly chopped garlic
- 1 28 ounce can crushed tasty tomatoes
- 1 10 ounce box of frozen corn
- 1 15 ½ ounce can of black beans (rinsed

well and drained)
- 1 cup of yellow cornmeal
- 1 cup of all-purpose flour
- 2 tablespoons of sugar
- 2 teaspoons of baking powder
- 1 teaspoon crystal salt
- 1/4 teaspoon of baking soda
- 1 cup of buttermilk
- 2 large eggs
- 6 tablespoons of unsalted butter (melted)
- 1/2 cup of thinly chopped scallion (green part only)

How to make

- Preheat the oven to 375 degrees Fahrenheit and lightly oil 7-8 ramekins.
- Take a 5- quart pot and heat the oil over moderately high temperature.
- Then add the turkey to the oil and cook. Next, break it up with a spoon while it is cooking. Then transfer the cooked turkey to a bowl.
- Put the onion in a pot and cook it until it becomes soft (about 3 minutes). Next, sprinkle the chili powder in the pot.
- Garlic should be added to the pot while stirring. Next, add in the tomatoes and all

the other ingredients, as well as the turkey.

- Then let it simmer about 10 minutes. Finally, remove the pan from the heat and add salt and pepper to taste.
- Take a bowl and whisk flour, baking soda, cornmeal, sugar, and salt. Then in another bowl, whisk together the buttermilk, eggs, and scallion.
- Now, take all the wet ingredients and slowly incorporate them into the dry ingredients.
- Then one cup of chili should be spooned into each arranged ramekin. Now you are going to want to top each ramekin of chili with cornbread and butter and it should be baked on a sheet pan.
- After that, it should be put in the oven. It should be baked about 25 minutes. The finished product will be golden brown color.

Fifth meal: hard boiled eggs and 2 whole crackers (wheat)

This meal supplies the body with the protein requirements and carbohydrate for the energy requirements of the body

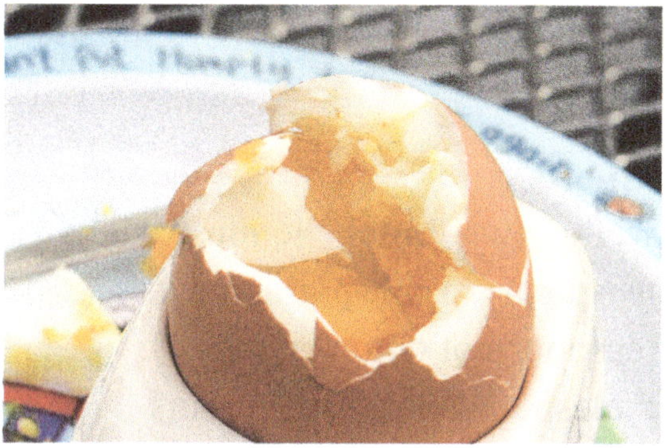

Sixth meal: Clean Eating Portobello Mushroom Burger

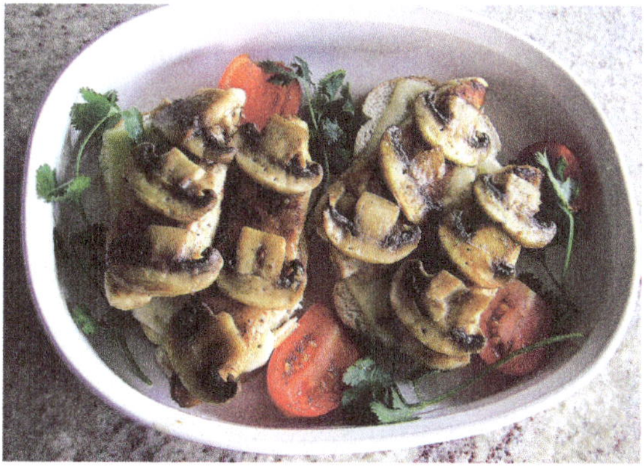

This is another delicious component of the clean eating process. This can be taken as the final meal of the day, so it should be tasty, as well as full of nutrients. This food has the appearance, as well as the taste of the traditional fast food.

Ingredients

- 4 well grown Portobello mushrooms
- 4 teaspoons of fine garlic powder
- 4 teaspoons of onion powder
- 8 tablespoons of alfalfa sprouts
- 4 tablespoons of ground avocado
- 4 teaspoons of mustard
- 4 fresh hamburger buns

How to make?

- Preheat the oven to 350o F
- Place the mushrooms on a parchment lined cookie sheet.
- Sprinkle onion powder and garlic powder on the mushrooms.
- Cover the cookie sheet with aluminum foil. Bake for about 20 minutes.
- Place mushroom on the bottom bun. Top with alfalfa sprouts, avocado, and spread the mustard on the top bun and place on top of the burger.

These meals are arranged according to the concepts of clean eating. The consumption of water should be about 3 liters. Water plays a comprehensive role in the process of clean eating, so it is better to have a higher amount of pure water than other types of beverages. The food items in the meal plan are very common and economical. They can be bought without paying a lot, and it is better to purchase directly from the farm itself.

The taste of certain food types on this list can be highly appreciated; this offers the total nutrition that a person should have. Although there is a long list of ingredients in the turkey and burger list, they are easy to find. The food items can be very useful to people who want to feed a family with children. The children love to enjoy these types of meals, as there are very delicious.

CHAPTER 6
-
Quick and simple clean eating recipes

The Clean Eating Diet is now becoming more and more popular around the globe. More people are now looking for recipes that will help them with their daily meal plans. The increase of demand on Clean Eating recipes are a good sign that many people are changing their eating habits and embracing the concept of going back to natural foods.

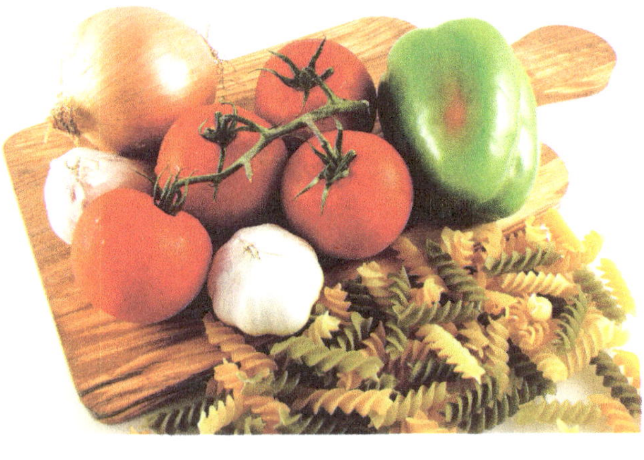

This proves to benefit mankind as a whole. In response to the demand of clean eating recipes, we have come up with 7 easy to prepare recipes that will fit anyone's budget. In this chapter you will find different recipes for breakfast, lunch, and dinner.

Breakfast

- Cheesy Potato Frittata
- Green Egg Skillet Bake
- Cherry Breakfast Rice Bowls

Lunch

- Orange Chicken Stir-Fry with Crispy Garlic Dressing
- Spaghetti Squash with Chicken, Pears, & Parmesan
- Greek-Style Grilled Fish with Cucumber Mint Yogurt

Dinner

- Quinoa salad
- Arugula, Grape, and Sunflower Seed Salad
- Tenderloin Steaks with Red Onion Marmalade

Breakfast Recipes

Cheesy Potato Frittata

This dish can be made with leftover potato wedges and has a creamy texture that is really delicious. This recipe is for 4 people, and a hand on time is 30 minutes. The total preparation time is 45 minutes.

Ingredients

- 8 fresh potatoes, scrubbed well and cut into 1/2-inch size cubes
- 1 large sized egg, plus 6 egg whites
- 2 tablespoons of skim milk
- 1/4 cup of finely sliced fresh parsley
- 1 tablespoon of ground fresh thyme
- 1/2 tablespoon of fresh and ground black pepper
- 1/2 tablespoon of sea salt, portioned.
- 1 tablespoon of safflower oil
- 1 1/2 cups of sliced yellow onion
- 1 clove garlic, minced
- 2 Oz of low-fat sharp cheddar cheese
- 1/2 cup of low fat sour cream (optional)

How to make?

- Bring 2 cups of water to a boil on medium high heat. Add potatoes and bring to boil. Boil for about 10 minutes. Drain the water and keep it aside.
- In a bowl, whisk egg, egg whites, milk, parsley, pepper, and 1/4 tablespoons of salt.

Set aside.

- Heat oil on medium high heat using a nonstick skillet. Add in onions; bring to cook while stirring now and then for about 6 minutes, or until the edges reach a light brown texture.
- Add garlic; bring to cook while stirring constantly for about 15 seconds. Add in potatoes, stir well until ingredients combine. Bring down the heat to medium low.
- Gently pour the egg mixture immediately over the top of potato mixture, distribute evenly. Cover the skillet and let it cook for 12 minutes.
- Once egg mixture is set, remove from heat. Sprinkle the remaining 1/4 tsp. of salt and cheddar.
- Let it sit for 15 minutes. Cut frittata into wedges and serve with sour cream and green onions.

Green Egg Skillet Bake

Ingredients

- 1 tablespoon of olive oil
- 1 white onion, thinly sliced
- 1/4 tablespoon of sea salt, plus a pinch

- Fresh ground black pepper, to taste
- 4 cups of roughly chopped collard greens
- 3 cloves garlic, minced, divided
- 1 tablespoon of ground cumin seeds
- 1/2 tablespoon of dried oregano
- 1/2 tablespoon of red pepper flakes
- 4 cups of roughly sliced spinach
- Some Olive oil cooking spray
- 5 white fresh mushrooms
- 4 large eggs
- 2 tablespoons of Greek yogurt
- 1 tablespoon 1% milk
- 2 tablespoons of red Chile paste

How to cook?

- Preheat the oven to 400°F.
- Place a large heavy bottomed pot over medium high heat. Add in oil and heat. Add onion first; stir-fry until it comes to a light brown texture, cooks in about 3 minutes. Add in salt, pepper, and collard greens.
- Let it cook while stirring, until it comes to a vibrant green texture, cooks for about 3 minutes. Add in 2 cloves garlic, cumin, oregano, and pepper flakes.
- Continue stirring to combine all ingredients together. Add in spinach. Let it cook while

continuously stirring. When spinach comes to a wilted texture, in about 2 minutes, remove from heat.

- Using the cooking spray, spray a cast iron skillet well. Remove the spinach mixture from the pot using tongs and transfer the mixture into the well-sprayed skillet. Leave excess liquid in the pot. Spread mushrooms over the top. In the spinach mixture, create 4 wells and crack the egg into the wells. Place in the oven and let it bake for about 8-10 minutes.
- While waiting for it to bake, whisk yogurt, milk, and remaining 1 clove garlic, and chili paste in a bowl. Spread the mixture in dollops on top of the spinach mixture.
- Serve with multigrain bread to soak up the egg yolks.

Cherry Breakfast Rice Bowls

Ingredients

- 1 cup of brown rice
- 1 tablespoon of safflower oil
- 2 tablespoons ground cinnamon
- 1/2 tablespoon of grated orange zest
- 1/4 tablespoon of sea salt

- 1/4 cup of skim milk
- 4 tablespoons of pure maple syrup
- 1/2 tablespoon of pure vanilla extract
- 1 packet of stevia
- 1 cup of frozen and unsweetened dark cherries

How to cook?

- Cook rice according to the instructions given, and mix with oil, orange zest, and salt. Then put into serving bowls.
- Take a small saucepan and bring milk and maple syrup to a boil, take off of the heat and stir in vanilla and stevia. Decorate the top of the rice mixture with the cherries.

Lunch Recipes

Orange Chicken Stir-Fry with Crispy Garlic Dressing

Ingredients

- 2/3 cup of brown rice
- 1 tablespoon of olive oil (should be divided)
- 7 1/2 oz. of BPA-free canned chickpeas, should be washed and dried
- 1/4 tablespoons of sea salt

- Cayenne pepper (ground)
- 1 bunch of broccoli (well-trimmed)
- 4 cloves of garlic, sliced very thinly
- 1 tablespoon of rice wine or apple cider vinegar
- 16 oz. of boneless, skinless chicken breasts (should be cut into 1-inch cubes)
- 1 zucchini, thinly sliced lengthwise
- 1 tablespoon of diluted -sodium soy sauce
- 1 tablespoon of ground ginger
- 1 peeled and divided orange. It should be cut into 1/2-inch cubes.
- 2 thinly sliced green onions

How to make?

- Cook rice according to directions.
- Take a large skillet and put 1 tablespoon of oil in the bottom. Add chickpeas and cook until they are golden in color. It will take about 15 minutes. Use salt and cayenne to season.
- Cook broccoli over a pot of simmering water for about 3 to 5 minutes. It should be cooked until the food is tender and crispy.
- Take a small saucepan and prepare the dressing. Heat oil and sauté the garlic let it

cook for about 4 minutes. Next, put it into a small dish and add some vinegar. Put it aside.

- Take another skillet. Heat the rest of the oil. Add chicken and sauté for about 5 minutes until it reaches medium heat. Next add zucchini, ginger, and soy sauce. It should be cooked about 5 to 7 minutes.

Spaghetti Squash with Chicken, Pears & Parmesan

Ingredients

- 3 pounds of spaghetti. It should be squashed, quartered, and seeded
- 1 tablespoon of olive oil
- 1-pound boneless and skinless chicken breasts, it should be cut into thick strips of ½ inch.
- 1 pear, cored and sliced
- 2 tablespoons of minced fresh chives
- 3 oz. Parmesan cheese

How to make?

Preheat the oven to 375°F. Put squash cut side up on a foil-lined, rimmed baking sheet. Pour in 1/4-inch water into the baking sheet. Bake until edges are golden brown. Pierce squash, if easily pierced with a fork or the tip of a knife then it is ready, cooks in about 35 minutes. Set aside and let cool enough to handle.

Using a large nonstick skillet, heat oil on medium heat, add chicken, and let it cook for about 2 minutes. Flip the chicken and add in pears and sage. Keep on stirring until chicken is cooked, cooks in about 5 minutes. Collect chicken, pears, and pan drippings into a large bowl.

Using 2 forks scrape off stringy squash flesh from the skin, having to separate it into strands. Add the squash flesh to bowl with the mixture of chicken. Add in chives, and toss to bring everything together. Top with cheese and serve.

Greek-Style Grilled Fish with Cucumber Mint Yogurt

Ingredients:

- 4 5-oz cod fillets
- 1/4 cup of 2% plain Greek yogurt
- 3 tablespoons of thinly chopped English cucumber
- 1 tablespoon of finely sliced fresh mint

leaves
- 1/2 green onion (chopped well)
- Sun flower cooking oil as needed
- 1/2 tablespoon of dried oregano
- 1/4 tablespoon and 1/8 tablespoon of sea salt, (in 2 parts)
- 1/4 tablespoon of fresh black pepper powder

How to make?
- Heat the outdoor grill with oil. Take the cod and sprinkle it with oregano, salt, and pepper powder and grill. It should be grilled for about 3 minutes.
- Meanwhile, in a small bowl, combine yogurt, cucumber, mint, onion, and remaining 1/8 tsp. salt. Serve with cod.
- Mix yoghurt, mint, onion, cucumber, and rest of the salt in another bowl and serve it with the grilled cod.

Dinner Recipes

Quinoa salad

Ingredients
- 1 teaspoon of olive oil
- 1/2 cup of finely sliced white onion
- 1 cup of uncooked quinoa

- 2 cups of pure water
- 1/2 teaspoon of kosher salt
- 1 cup of fresh orange sections (must have one large orange)
- 1/4 cup of chopped pecans, (should be toasted)
- 2 tablespoons of onion (minced)
- 5 dates, sliced
- 1/2 pound of (2-inch) slices of asparagus

For Dressing:

- 2 tablespoons of fresh lemon juice
- 1 tablespoon of olive oil
- 1/4 teaspoon of kosher salt
- 1/4 teaspoon freshly ground black pepper
- 1 garlic clove
- 2 tablespoons of freshly chopped mint

How to make?

- Take a nonstick saucepan and heat the oil over medium high heat. Add in white onion and let it sauté about 2 minutes.
- Add the quinoa, 2 cups of water, and ½ teaspoon of salt to the pan. Then bring to a boil. Let it simmer for about 15 minutes after covering.
- Take it off of the heat and let it rest. It will

take about 15 minutes. Place the mixture of quinoa in another bowl.
- Add orange and rest of the ingredients and toss it to become more compound.
- Then next step is the preparation of the dressing. Mix juice and other 4 ingredients in a medium bowl, then stir well, and pour the dressing over the salad, mix gently, and for added flavor, it can be sprinkled with mint.

Arugula, Grape, and Sunflower Seed Salad

Ingredients
- 3 tablespoons of red wine vinegar
- 1 teaspoon of honey
- 1 teaspoon of pure maple syrup
- 1/2 teaspoon of ground mustard
- 2 teaspoons of grape seed oil
- 7 cups of loosely packed baby arugula
- 2 cups of red grapes
- 2 tablespoons of sunflower seed kernels (toasted)
- 1 teaspoon of chopped fresh thyme
- 1/4 teaspoon of salt
- 1/4 teaspoon of freshly black pepper powder

How to make?

- Take a bowl and mix vinegar, syrup, honey, and mustard. Then whisk in oil.
- Take a large bowl and mix arugula, seeds, grapes, and thyme. Drizzle the dressing over the arugula. Then add salt and pepper to taste.

Tenderloin Steaks with Red Onion Marmalade

Ingredients

- 1 large red onion should be sliced and separated into rings (2 cups)
- 2 tablespoons of red wine vinegar
- 2 tablespoons of honey
- 1/2 teaspoon of salt of portioned
- 1 teaspoon of dried thyme
- 1/4 teaspoon of fresh black pepper powder
- 4 oz. of beef tenderloin steaks, trimmed

How to cook?

- Preheat the broiler to relevant temperature.
- Heat a large nonstick saucepan over medium high heat. Spray the pan with cooking oil. Then add in an onion and cook about 3

minutes.

- Add vinegar, 1/4 teaspoon of salt, and honey in the pan. Next, decrease the heat and let it simmer.
- Uncover the pan, and let it become slightly thick. It should be stirred now and then.
- Put rest of the salt, thyme, and pepper over the beef, then put it in the broiler and for about 4 minutes for each side. It is nice to serve with onion rings.

CONCLUSION

As a result of clean eating, beautiful changes in the human body are noticeable, a slim and firm body, no bulges, and just the right body weight. Constant food supply meets the total energy requirements of the body, thus, making the person energetic and non-sluggish.

Water in every aspect is important for people to live. The human body alone cannot survive without water. It is, therefore, imperative to nourish the body with lots of water along with clean eating to keep it healthy and strengthen the immune system. The daily requirement of water must be at least 8 glasses of water or beyond.

The supply of important vitamins and other nutrients help improve the condition of skin and hair. A balanced diet and the right amount of nutrients offer positive development in the relaxation of the body, so the person can enjoy long and peaceful sleep. In general, clean eating is important to keep the appearance of a person in its best form. It makes a person younger and healthier.

ABOUT THE AUTHOR

Barbara Neil's desire to help others avoid a life of obesity is what encouraged her to write books about clean living and healthy foods. In her younger years, Barbara had her fair share of health issues in terms of weight and obesity. Many of the issues she faced could have been avoided if only she was properly educated about the dangers of fast food diets. In her desire to lose weight and slim down, she went through crash diets that made her situation turn from bad to worse.

She went through thorough research and came to the realization that she needed to go back to the basics and change her eating habits. Her family and friends supported her throughout her journey while she became very serious about the foods she should take in and foods that she should not. She later on developed a clean eating diet that proves to be healthy and good for the body.

Her research along with advice from her doctors and support from her family and friends,

Barbara was able to lose all the excess weight, slim down, and look good. It all boils down to changing the way she looked at food. Her life was transformed just about instantly. From a loser to a winner, she is now able to fit in and really feel confident about herself. Barbara hopes that through her books, she will be able to influence young men and women to change their eating habits and live a happy and healthy life that promises a lot of benefits.

Lightning Source UK Ltd.
Milton Keynes UK
UKOW06f2305060715

254678UK00011BA/69/P

9 781634 283496